My Life Has a Story

A Guided Autobiography

By

Amy Brennan

ISBN: 1-4107-3265-7 (e-book)
ISBN: 1-4107-3266-5 (Paperback)

Library of Congress Control Number: 2003092369

This book is printed on acid free paper.

Printed in the United States of America
Bloomington, IN

1stBooks – rev. 07/16/03

In memory of Uncle Don, who was the

reason I started this project,

and for my friend Etta, who is more

alive now than she was 40 years ago.

Instructions

This book is about you. It is not intended to be a complete autobiography, but rather an outline of some of the major aspects of your life and experiences.

Feel free to fill in pages in any order you choose, add details or stories in the extra space, skip over questions, copy pages, take out pages you do not need, and add pages of your own.

One thing should be stressed—do not be humble. You may find yourself wondering why anyone would ever want to know such silly or insignificant facts. Details about your life are not insignificant; they make you who you are.

Lastly, and perhaps most importantly, share your story with someone. You do not need to have filled in every blank, nor have every *i* dotted and *t* crossed. The people who love you already know you are not perfect!

Make this book your own. Dig up old memories. Share your opinions and advice. Give someone a piece of your life story.

The Basics

Full name _____

I was given this name because _____

Date of birth _____

Place of birth _____

Places I have lived _____

Spouse's name(s) _____

Children's names _____

_____

Parents' names _____

Brothers' and/or sisters' names _____

_____

Grandparents' names_____

My height is _____

My hair color is _____

My hair color at 30 was _____

My weight is _____

My approximate weight at 30 was _____

My eye color is _____

Favorites

Catch phrase _____

Nickname for myself_____

Kind of music _____

Song_____

Book _____

Magazine _____

Piece of art _____

Movie _____

Movie star_____

TV show _____

Anchorperson_____

Radio station _____

Card game _____

Board game _____

Color_____

Flower_____

Musical instrument _____

Restaurant _____

Fast food restaurant_____

Food _____

Snack food _____

Dessert_____

Ice cream flavor _____

More Favorites

Drink _____

Soda _____

Smell _____

Sound _____

Fabric or texture _____

Time of day _____

Time of year _____

Kind of weather _____

Vacation spot _____

Holiday _____

Holiday food _____

Holiday song _____

Car I ever owned _____

Outfit I ever wore _____

Prized possession _____

Cause or charity _____

Family

One non-holiday tradition my family had was_____

_____

For my birthday when I was young, my family usually _____

_____

At dinnertime when I was young, my family usually _____

_____

When there was food on my plate I didn't want to eat, my parents usually _____

My mother's main role with the children was _____

_____

My father's main role with the children was _____

_____

The "favorite" in my family was_____

The family member that I had an especially close bond with was_____

The family member that I never quite saw eye to eye with was

_____

One household chore I didn't mind doing was _____

_____

My least favorite household chore was _____

Mother and Father

I would describe my mother and father's marriage as _____

_____

One thing that keeps/kept my mother and father together is/was _____

_____

One way my parents are/were very different is/was_____

_____

_____

One memorable occasion my parents got dressed up for was

_____

_____

The best gift I remember my father buying for my mother was

_____

_____

The thing I admire(d) most about them was_____

_____

_____

My mother is/lived to be _____ years old.

My father is/lived to be _____ years old.

Mother

Name _____

Birth date _____

I called her _____

The nickname she had for me was _____

Two words to describe her as a parent are _____

_____

Two words to describe her as a person are _____

_____

I would describe our relationship as _____

_____

I think she would have described our relationship when I was
under her roof as _____

_____

I think she would describe our relationship after I became an
adult as _____

_____

One of the best memories I have with her is _____

_____

One thing that I would want her to forget about me is _____

_____

The one thing I want to tell her is _____

_____

Another woman that I viewed as a mother figure in my life

is/was _____

_____

_____

_____

_____

_____

_____

_____

_____

_____

_____

_____

_____

_____

_____

_____

Father

Name _____

Birth date _____

I called him _____

The nickname he had for me was _____

Two words to describe him as a parent are _____

_____

Two words to describe him as a person are_____

_____

I would describe our relationship as_____

_____

I think he would have described our relationship when I was under his roof as_____

_____

I think he would describe our relationship after I became an adult as_____

_____

One of the best memories I have with him is _____

_____

One thing that I would want him to forget about me is _____

_____

The one thing I want to tell him is _____

_____

Another man I viewed as a father figure in my life is/was _____

_____

_____

_____

_____

_____

_____

_____

_____

_____

_____

_____

_____

_____

_____

_____

Brothers and Sisters

I am the (oldest, youngest, etc.) _____ child.

One way people can tell I am related to my sibling(s) is

_____

One way I am completely different from my sibling(s) is

_____

When we were younger, I took the blame for something that was not my fault when _____

_____

When we were younger, one of my siblings took the blame for me when_____

_____

One time I was very happy to have brothers and/or sisters was

_____

_____

If I had been an only child, my life would have been different because _____

_____

Brother/Sister #1

Name _____

Birth date _____

Two words to describe him/her as a child or teenager are ___

_____

I would describe our relationship as_____

_____

I think he/she would describe our relationship as_____

_____

One of the best memories I have with him/her is _____

_____

_____

I am most proud of my brother/sister because_____

_____

_____

Brother/Sister #2

Name _____

Birth date _____

Two words to describe him/her as a child or teenager are ____

_____

I would describe our relationship as _____

_____

I think he/she would describe our relationship as_____

_____

One of the best memories I have with him/her is _____

_____

_____

I am most proud of my brother/sister because_____

_____

_____

Brother/Sister #___

(Copy this page if more are needed)

Name _____

Birth date _____

Two words to describe him/her as a child or teenager are ___

_____

I would describe our relationship as_____

_____

I think he/she would describe our relationship as_____

_____

One of the best memories I have with him/her is _____

_____

_____

I am most proud of my brother/sister because_____

_____

_____

Grandparents

In my life, I got to know (how many) _____ of my grandparents.

Maternal Grandparents

The two words that best describe my maternal grandparents are _____

_____

My mother would say the two words that best describe her parents are _____

_____

_____

My father would say the two words that best describe his in-laws are _____

_____

_____

The funniest story I ever heard about one of my maternal grandparents is_____

_____

_____

If I could ask my maternal grandparents one question about my mother, it would be _____

_____

When I think of my maternal grandparents, I think of the smells of _____

and _____

_____

_____

_____

_____

_____

_____

_____

_____

_____

_____

_____

_____

_____

Paternal Grandparents

The two words that best describe my paternal grandparents are _____

_____

My father would say the two words that best describe his parents are _____

_____

My mother would say the two words that best describe her in-laws are _____

_____

The funniest story I ever heard about one of my paternal grandparents is_____

_____

_____

If I could ask my paternal grandparents one question about my father, it would be_____

_____

When I think of my paternal grandparents, I think of the smells of _____

and _____

Marriage

The first time I met my husband/wife, we were (place)

_____

The first time I met my husband/wife, I remember thinking ____

_____

On our first date, we went _____

I proposed/was proposed to (when)_____

(where) _____

When we told my family, the reaction was _____

_____

When we told his/her family, the reaction was _____

_____

We had known each other for _____

before we got married. I was _____ years old.

We married on (date) _____

On my wedding day, I felt_____

Something special I remember from my wedding day is

_____

We went on our honeymoon to _____

We lived (where) _____

One of the worst fights we ever had was about _____

_____

We worked through it by _____

My husband/wife is/was very good at taking care of_____

_____

We were/have been married _____ years.

_____

_____

_____

_____

_____

_____

_____

_____

_____

_____

_____

_____

_____

Re-Marriage

The first time I met my second husband/wife, I remember thinking _____

On our first date, we went _____

I proposed/was proposed to (when)_____

(where) _____

The biggest lesson I learned from my first marriage was_____

_____

The biggest thing I knew I still needed to work on was _____

_____

We had known each other for _____ before we got

married. I was _____ years old.

We married on (date) _____

On my wedding day, I felt_____

Something special I remember from my wedding day is _____

_____

We went on our honeymoon to _____

We lived (where) _____

One of the worst fights we ever had was about _____

_____

We worked through it by _____

My husband/wife is/was very good at taking care of_____

_____

We were/have been married _____ years.

_____

_____

_____

_____

_____

_____

_____

_____

_____

_____

_____

_____

_____

_____

_____

Children

I have _____ child/children.

When I found out I was going to be a mother/father for the first time, I felt _____

My main role with my child/children is/was_____

_____

My spouse's main role with our child/children is/was_____

_____

My favorite age of a child is _____

because _____

As my child/children got older, my biggest challenge was _____

_____

When my first child left the house, I felt _____

_____

When my last child left the house, I felt _____

_____

One specific time I felt incredibly happy to be a parent was ___

_____

One specific time I felt incredibly scared to be a parent was ___

_____

_____

Child #1

Name _____

He/She was given that name because_____

_____

He/She was born on (date) _____

in (place)_____

Two words to describe him/her as a child or teenager are ___

_____

Two words to describe him/her as an adult are _____

_____

One thing I would have liked to change as a parent was_____

_____

One of my favorite stories to tell about him/her is _____

_____

_____

One of the best memories I have with him/her is _____

_____

_____

I am most proud of my son/daughter because_____

_____

_____

Child #2

Name _____

He/She was given that name because _____

_____

He/She was born on (date) _____

in (place)_____

Two words to describe him/her as a child or teenager are ___

_____

Two words to describe him/her as an adult are _____

_____

One thing I would have liked to change as a parent was_____

_____

One of my favorite stories to tell about him/her is _____

_____

_____

One of the best memories I have with him/her is_____

_____

_____

I am most proud of my son/daughter because_____

_____

_____

Child #____

(Copy this page if more pages are needed)

Name _____

He/She was given that name because_____

_____

He/She was born on (date) _____

in (place)_____

Two words to describe him/her as a child or teenager are ____

_____

Two words to describe him/her as an adult are _____

_____

One thing I would have liked to change as a parent was_____

_____

One of my favorite stories to tell about him/her is _____

_____

One of the best memories I have with him/her is _____

_____

I am most proud of my son/daughter because_____

_____

Grandchildren

I have _____ grandchild/grandchildren.

When I found out I was going to be a grandparent for the first time, I felt _____

I think my primary role as a grandparent is _____

_____

One thing that my mother or father did for my children that I want to do for my grandchildren is _____

_____

One thing that my mother or father did for my children that I do not want to do for my grandchildren is _____

_____

One thing that one of my grandchildren did that reminded me of his/her mother or father was_____

_____

If I could give my child/children one piece of advice about parenting, it would be _____

_____

The thing I most enjoy about being a grandparent is_____

_____

Friends

The friend I have known the longest that I still keep in touch with is _____

We have known each other _____ years.

One person I wish I had kept in better touch with is/was _____

_____

One person who I became friends with despite our differences is/was _____

One person who I became friends with because of our similarities is/was _____

One person that I am surprised to hear from/about every once in a while is/was _____

In my opinion, the definition of a friend is_____

_____

_____

Friend #1

Name _____

I met this friend _____ years ago.

We met (how)_____

Two words I would use to describe him/her as a person would

be _____

Two words I think he/she would use to describe me are _____

_____

As a friend, he/she is/was good at _____

_____

If I could apologize to this friend for one thing, it would be ____

_____

One of the best memories I have with him/her is _____

_____

_____

Friend #2

Name _____

I met this friend _____ years ago.

We met (how)_____

Two words I would use to describe him/her as a person would

be _____

Two words I think he/she would use to describe me are _____

_____

As a friend, he/she is/was good at _____

_____

If I could apologize to this friend for one thing, it would be ____

_____

One of the best memories I have with him/her is _____

_____

_____

Friend #____

(Copy this page if more pages are needed)

Name _____

I met this friend _____ years ago.

We met (how)_____

Two words I would use to describe him/her as a person would

be _____

Two words I think he/she would use to describe me are _____

_____

As a friend, he/she is/was good at _____

_____

If I could apologize to this friend for one thing, it would be ____

_____

One of the best memories I have with him/her is_____

_____

_____

Pets

In my life, I have had_____ pets.

As a child, my favorite pet was a _____

named _____

The day I had to say goodbye to that pet, I felt _____

_____

One animal I always wanted as a pet was a _____

_____

One type of animal I had as a pet once, and never want as a

pet again is _____

As an adult, my favorite pet is/was a _____

named _____

This animal loves/loved to _____

_____

What makes/made me happiest about this pet is/was_____

_____

_____

Childhood

My earliest memory of my life is _____

My first best friend was _____

I was taught to read by _____

I was taught how to tie my shoes by _____

My favorite playground game was _____

I remember being teased by _____

because _____

I remember teasing _____

because _____

I enjoyed the_____ grade the most because _____

_____

My favorite elementary school teacher was _____

My favorite toys or games were _____

The friend I enjoyed playing with the most was _____

When I was sick, my parents would _____

_____

When I was scared, my parents would_____

_____

The first person I had a crush on was _____

Teen Years

My first kiss was from _____

My first real boyfriend or girlfriend was _____

The last time I heard about that person, he/she was _____

_____

My first car was _____

My best friend(s) was/were _____

_____

I liked to go out with my friends and _____

My favorite hangout was _____

The subject I did the best in was _____

because _____

The subject I did the worst in was _____

because _____

The club or activity I enjoyed being a part of the most was ____

_____

My favorite teacher was _____

My overall impression of school was _____

My first job was_____

I mainly used my paychecks to pay for _____

I used to get in trouble for_____

I made my parents proud when_____

I graduated in (year) _____

If I knew then what I know now, I would have_____

_____

_____

_____

_____

_____

_____

_____

_____

_____

_____

_____

_____

_____

_____

_____

_____

_____

Early Adulthood

I left my parents' house at the age of _____

I left because _____

I was working/going to school at _____

My first place on my own, with a roommate, or with my spouse

was _____

One on the first big problems I had to take care of on my own

was _____

_____

The hardest lesson I learned about entering the "real world"

was _____

_____

_____

Military Duty

The branch of the military I serve(d) in is/was _____

_____

My reason for joining the military was _____

_____

I joined in (year) _____ at the age of _____

My military duties (stations and tours) include(d)_____

_____

_____

The highest rank I received is _____

Military honors and awards I received include _____

_____

My most memorable commanding officer was_____

_____

I was discharged/retired after _____ years.

One thing that my military service taught me is _____

_____

If I could say one thing about patriotism, it would be _____

_____

College

The name of the college or university I attended is _____

_____

I chose to attend this school because _____

_____

While attending this college, I lived (where)_____

_____

My major was _____

If I had the chance to do it over again, I might have majored in

_____

Activities I was involved in included _____

_____

One memorable tradition I took part in was _____

_____

One mischievous thing my friends and I did was_____

_____

One class I enjoyed attending was_____

One class I had a hard time with was_____

because _____

_____

During my college years, I worked hard at _____

_____

During my college years, I could have spent more time working

on _____

On graduation day, I felt _____

_____

_____

_____

_____

_____

_____

_____

_____

_____

_____

_____

_____

_____

_____

Work

When I was young, I wanted to be _____

I started working when I was (age)_____

My first job was_____

The most important lesson I learned from my first job was ___

_____

My favorite job was_____

My least favorite job was _____

My best work habit is/was _____

My worst work habit is/was_____

The best piece of advice I ever got from a boss was_____

_____

One job I always thought I would be good at is _____

If I could get paid to _____

all day, that is what I would do.

One of my favorite co-workers was _____

One of my favorite bosses was _____

I remember thinking I had done pretty well for myself when __

_____

I retired in (year)_____

from _____

Home

My favorite house I have ever lived in is/was_____

_____

One item I always like to have prominently placed in my home

is_____

My favorite color/texture for the exterior of a house is _____

_____

I would describe my decorating taste as _____

One of the biggest renovations I ever undertook on my house

was_____

One of the biggest disasters I ever had happen to my house

was_____

One trait that makes a house feel "homey" is_____

_____

My favorite place to sit and relax in my current home is _____

_____

In nice weather, the place I like to spend my time is _____

_____

In poor weather, the place I like to spend my time is _____

_____

I love when my house smells like_____

Appearance

Distinguishing marks (scars, birthmarks, tattoos) I have include

_____

_____

The age at which I look/looked the best is/was _____

The biggest physical change I ever noticed in myself was ____

_____

My most flattering feature is my _____

One feature I wish I could change is _____

I think I look my best when _____

I think I look my worst when _____

One color of clothing that suits me is _____

One color of clothing that does not suit me is _____

One item I always carry with me is_____

One article of clothing I dislike shopping for is _____

_____

I would describe the style of my appearance as _____

_____

One physical characteristic I find attractive in the opposite sex

is_____

Hobbies and Leisure

My favorite pastime is_____

When I am doing this, I feel _____

The most creative thing I have ever made is _____

_____

One thing I want to invent is_____

_____

One thing I collect/used to collect is/was _____

_____

When I want to relax, I _____

Clubs and organizations I am a member of include_____

_____

One thing I like to do outdoors is _____

One thing I enjoy about nature is _____

One thing I do not enjoy about nature is _____

_____

One physical activity I enjoy taking part in is _____

_____

If I could describe "shopping" in one word it would be

_____

My favorite store to shop at is _____

because _____

The brand names I am loyal to are _____

_____

_____

_____

_____

_____

_____

_____

_____

_____

_____

_____

_____

_____

_____

_____

Travel

When I was young, one memorable place my family went was

_____

One time I felt a little homesick was _____

_____

The first time I rode in a train was _____

_____

The first time I flew in an airplane was _____

_____

The farthest from home I have ever been is _____

_____

One place I have visited that I was happy to return home from

was _____

One place I have visited that I would like to move to is _____

_____

One vacation spot I have no interest in going to is _____

_____

One vacation spot I would like to go to is _____

_____

When I am on vacation, some things I like to do are _____

_____

Entertainment

The first movie I remember seeing in the theater was _____

_____

One movie that had a big impact on me was _____

because _____

One movie that made me laugh was _____

One movie that made me cry was _____

One Hollywood tragedy I remember is _____

_____

One band or singer I saw perform that I enjoyed was _____

_____

One song that made me laugh was _____

One song that made me cry was _____

One radio program I enjoy/enjoyed listening to is/was_____

_____

One type of cultural event I enjoy seeing live on stage is _____

_____

The most memorable stage show I have seen is_____

_____

I think the person who has made the greatest contribution to entertainment is_____

because_____

If I had to chance to be a part of the entertainment world, I would enjoy being _____

_____

_____

_____

_____

_____

_____

_____

_____

_____

_____

_____

_____

_____

_____

Sports

My favorite sport is _____

My least favorite sport is_____

I am loyal to _____

The team I dislike the most is_____

On a scale of 1 – 10, I would rate my level of enthusiasm for

this team at_____

I started rooting for this team when I was (age)_____

because _____

One of the most exciting games I have ever seen was when _

_____

One game that was a big disappointment was when_____

_____

The food that best accompanies watching this sport/team is__

_____

Politics and World Events

My political affiliation is_____

because _____

My favorite president is/was_____

because _____

My least favorite political figure is/was_____

because _____

The historical figure that I admire the most is_____

because _____

One political ideal I strongly support/supported is/was

_____

The event in my community that has had the greatest impact

on me is _____

because _____

The world event that has had the greatest impact on me is____

_____

When this event happened, I felt _____

_____

_____

Social Issues

One major problem in society that I think needs to be fixed is_

_____

One example of the fallibility of the human race is_____

One example of a great act of human kindness is_____

Comment briefly on the following issues:

Civil rights_____

Education _____

Freedom of speech _____

Healthcare _____

Homelessness _____

Immigration_____

Military intervention _____

Prejudice _____

Single parenthood _____

Social Security _____

Taxes _____

Treatment of the elderly _____

Unemployment_____

Welfare_____

Religion

I would describe my religious beliefs as _____

_____

My religious affiliation is _____

My favorite passage from scripture is_____

_____

My favorite spiritual song is _____

My place of worship is _____

The thing I like best about my place of worship is _____

_____

Spiritually, I feel that my beliefs offer me _____

_____

One time that I feel my beliefs were tested was when _____

_____

One time that my beliefs helped me persevere was when_____

_____

_____

Me

One thing that can always make me laugh is_____

_____

I think I am very good at_____

I think I am not very good at_____

My least favorite household chore is _____

My favorite household chore is_____

I am afraid of _____

Something I always need help with is _____

_____

Something I can usually help others with is _____

_____

If I could go back and do something over again, it would be __

_____

_____

The most important thing in my life is_____

_____

One thing I don't like about getting older is _____

_____

One thing I love about getting older is _____

_____

Memories

The best gift I ever received was _____

_____

The best vacation I ever took was _____

_____

The most memorable birthday I ever had was _____

_____

The most memorable anniversary I ever had was _____

_____

The worst habit I ever kicked was _____

The worst habit I still have is _____

The biggest heartbreak I ever had was _____

_____

_____

The most exciting change I ever made in my life was _____

_____

_____

One of the most exciting events I ever took part in was _____

_____

_____

The thing about me that I think would most impress my grandchildren is_____

_____

The goal I am most proud of achieving in my life is _____

_____

The goal that I still want to achieve is _____

_____

_____

_____

_____

_____

_____

_____

_____

_____

_____

_____

_____

_____

_____

More Memories

The most famous person I have ever met was _____

_____

One of my most embarrassing moments was _____

_____

The worst injury I ever sustained was _____

_____

The biggest run-in with the law I ever had was _____

_____

I laughed the hardest I have ever laughed when _____

_____

I cried the hardest I have ever cried when _____

_____

I felt the most scared I have ever felt when _____

_____

I felt the most content I have ever felt when_____

_____

One person I would like to thank for how much they affected my life is _____

The best time of my life is/was _____

In My Lifetime...

When I was born, the president was _____

Major world events that have happened in my lifetime include

_____

_____

Major medical advancements that have happened include ____

_____

Major transportation improvements that have taken place include _____

_____

Major technological advancements that have been invented include _____

_____

Major changes that have affected our everyday lives include _

_____

The most ridiculous invention I have seen is _____

_____

The most useful invention I have seen is _____

_____

Advice

The best piece of advice anyone ever gave me was _____

_____

_____

_____

If I could give one piece of advice about money, it would be __

_____

_____

_____

If I could give one piece of advice about love, it would be _____

_____

_____

_____

If I could give one piece of advice about friendships, it would

be _____

_____

_____

If I could give one piece of advice about life in general, it would

be _____

_____

_____

Circle or underline your preference.

scrambled	or	fried
creamy	or	crunchy
vanilla	or	chocolate
ham	or	turkey
coffee	or	tea
cream	or	sugar
red apples	or	yellow apples
blinds	or	curtains
elevator	or	stairs
automatic	or	manual
white walls in	or	white walls out
cash	or	credit
individual stocks	or	mutual funds
telephone call	or	letter
going out to dinner	or	eating at home
hotel	or	motel
driving on vacation	or	flying on vacation
being in the spotlight	or	being behind the scenes
theater	or	movies
dogs	or	cats
dressing up	or	dressing down
socks	or	slippers
talking	or	listening
big cities	or	small towns
paint	or	wallpaper
a busy day	or	a lazy day
naiveté and youth	or	age and experience

About the Author

Amy Brennan grew up in Indiana, and earned an English degree from Butler University in Indianapolis. She worked in the publishing industry for several years in Phoenix, Arizona, before changing careers and becoming a teacher. Amy is currently living and working in Japan with her husband, Paul. This is her first book.

www.ingramcontent.com/pod-product-compliance
Lightning Source LLC
Chambersburg PA
CBHW080421290526
45791CB00008BA/2367